YOUR KNOWLEDGE HAS VALUE

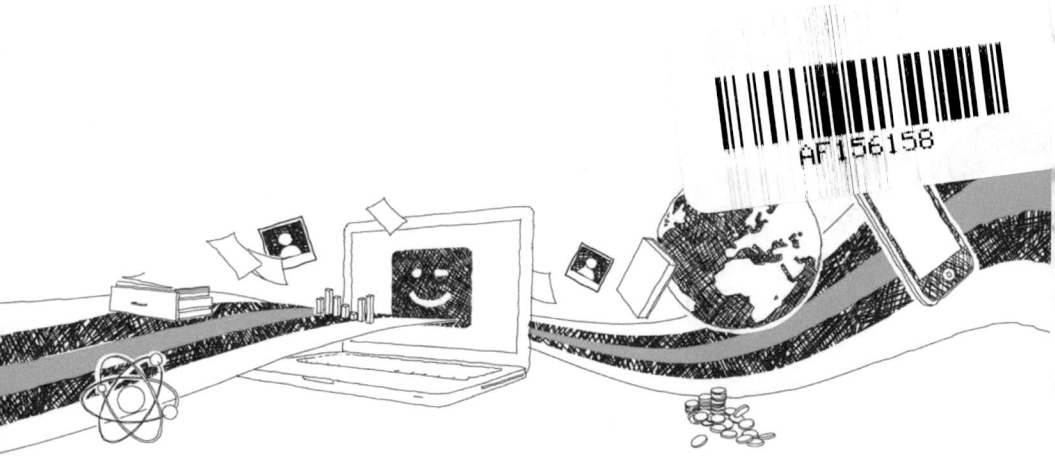

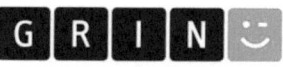

Bibliographic information published by the German National Library:

The German National Library lists this publication in the National Bibliography; detailed bibliographic data are available on the Internet at http://dnb.dnb.de .

Imprint:

Copyright © 2019 GRIN Verlag
Print and binding: Books on Demand GmbH, Norderstedt Germany
ISBN: 9783346167347

This book at GRIN:

https://www.grin.com/document/540380

Stefan G. Raul

Aus der Reihe: e-fellows.net stipendiaten-wissen

e-fellows.net (Hrsg.)

Band 3382

Policy issue: Alcohol consumption in Germany

GRIN Verlag

GRIN - Your knowledge has value

Since its foundation in 1998, GRIN has specialized in publishing academic texts by students, college teachers and other academics as e-book and printed book. The website www.grin.com is an ideal platform for presenting term papers, final papers, scientific essays, dissertations and specialist books.

Visit us on the internet:

http://www.grin.com/

http://www.facebook.com/grincom

http://www.twitter.com/grin_com

EMPA - CII-1: Policy Making: Actors, Institutions and Processes

Academic Year 2019/2020

Assignment # 2: essay

Due on: Monday, November 4th 2019, 10 pm

Topic of the essay: **Alcohol consumption in Germany**

Student: Stefan Raul

I

Table of contents

List of illustrations and figures II

List of abbreviations II

Referencing details II

1 Intro 1

2 Most critical governance challenges 2

3 Weakest points of existing interventions 6

4 Delegation of authority 8

Bibliography III

List of illustrations and figures

Figure 1 - Direct cost related to harmful alcohol consumption 4

Figure 2 - Indirect cost related to harmful alcohol consumption 5

List of abbreviations

BGB	Bürgerliches Gesetzbuch (German civil code)
BKiSchG	Bundeskinderschutzgesetz (Federal Child Protection Act)
bn	Billion
BSI	Bundesverband der Deutschen Spirituosen-Industrie und -Import-eure e.V. (German association for the spirits industry and importers)
BZgA	Bundeszentrale für gesundheitliche Aufklärung (Federal Center for Health Education)
CNAPA	Committee on National Alcohol Policy and Action
DKFZ	Deutsches Krebsforschungszentrum (German Cancer Research Institute)
EAHF	European Alcohol and Health Forum
EU	European Union
EUR	Euro
JuSchG	Jugendschutzgesetz (Protection of Young Persons Act)
p.a.	per annum

Referencing details

This document is written in reference to the APA style, regarding citations. The basis for this style was taken from the document 'A quick Hertie School Library guide for EMPA students', provided by Hertie School in September 2019 (Hertie School, 2019, pp. 19).

1 Intro

In Germany, 99.0 million hectoliters of alcoholic beverages were sold in the year of 2016 (Schaller et al., 2017, pp. 36). Although the per capita consumption of alcohol has dropped in the last 40 years in Germany, compared internationally, it continues to be one of the high-consumption countries in the world (Drogenbeauftragte der Bundesregierung, 2018, p. 56). Addictions are societal challenges that require the interaction of all social forces in the interest of the affected people (Drogenbeauftragte der Bundesregierung, 2018, p. 9).

The essay tries to consider the most critical governance challenges involved in tackling the issue[1], looks at the possibly weakest points of existing interventions vis-à-vis the problem and does a quick check of arguments for and against delegating authority to the supranational level.

---

[1] There is a thin line between regular alcohol consumption and harmful alcohol consumption. As there is no final and agreed upon definition to when alcohol is harmful for an individual (Singer and Teyssen, 2001, URL), the assumption within the essay is that there is no specific differentiation between these two fields.

2 Most critical governance challenges

When looking into the topic of governance challenges, the first step is to understand what governance is. According to the World Bank, governance is the "manner in which power is exercised in the management of a country's economic and social resources for development" (World Bank, 1991, in Anheier, 2013, p. 16). In a more detailed view, governance orders and dimensions can be distinguished. In first-order governance, it is about politics and the dimensions include legitimacy and a public problem, meaning that the main tasks include defining the basis of power and the allocation of rights and responsibilities as well as the definition and framing of the public problem. In second-order governance it is about policies and the dimensions include institutions and organizations as well as regulation and control. The main tasks include the setting of rules and the monitoring and sanctioning inherent to regulating and controlling an issue. In the gorvernance order of the policy outcome, it is about the performance, meaning that if a goal was attained or not (Kooiman and Jentoft, 2009, in Anheier, 2013, pp. 16).

When considering the most critical governance challenges to tackle the issue regarding the consumption of alcohol in Germany, for this essay, three major topics are in the center of attention.[2]

The first one of the three topics is the availability of alcohol, especially the advertising of products regarding alcohol. The second topic is the possibility of raising the legal drinking age to 18 years, implying a prohibition of the consumption of alcohol at a younger age. The third topic is the reduction of economic damage caused by alcohol consumption, which shall also be a goal of effective governance when tackling the issue.

Advertising of products regarding alcohol

There is regional legislation in each federal state which prohibits or restricts the promotion of alcoholic beverages in various media. In addition, the spirits industry takes its responsibility for the presentation and promotion of alcohol in the form of self-regulation (BSI, 2019, URL). The basis of this self-commitment policy is a Code of Conduct for the 'commercial communication of alcoholic beverages' which was presented in 2009 by the

---

[2] Different sources were screened and for this essay, three focus topics were selected (Singer and Teyssen, 2001, URL; Young, 2017, URL; „Deutschland hat ein Alkoholproblem", 2019, URL).

Deutscher Werberat (German Advertising Council)³. This Code of Conduct includes amongst other content the self-regulation policy to prevent representations or statements in the commercial communication for products as an invitation to the abusive consumption of alcohol as well as the assurance that the legal provisions in the field of commercial communication for alcoholic beverages are respected (Deutscher Werberat, 2015, p. 4).

The governance challenge for this topic lies in second-order governance, in the dimension of regulation and control. This is due to the fact that the monitoring of compliance with this Code of Conduct, the organization of the complaint procedure and the assessment are the responsibility of the German Advertising Council (Deutscher Werberat, 2015, p. 4).

Raising the legal drinking age to 18 years
Differentiating between private and public space, the former has no specific legal restriction with regard to underage drinking, but parents in general are obliged to care for and protect their children, according to the *Bundeskinderschutzgesetz* (Federal Child Protection Act, abbreviated: BKiSchG). Within the public space, the purchase and the consumption of alcohol is regulated via the *Jugendschutzgesetz* (Protection of Young Persons Act, abbreviated: JuSchG), especially in § 9 of the JuSchG.

According to § 9 JuSchG section 2 and § 1 JuSchG section 1 no. 2, minors under age 16 (specifically at age 14) are allowed to consume (undistilled) alcoholic beverages e.g. beer and wine when they are accompanied by a custodial person. According to § 9 JuSchG section 1 no. 2, minors at age 16 are allowed to consume (undistilled) alcoholic beverages without a custodial person or parent. At the age of 18, when people in Germany legally become adults⁴, they are allowed to access and consume distilled spirits and alcoholic beverages, according to § 9 JuSchG section 1 no. 1.

Although the alcohol consumption among adolescents has fallen by about two-thirds since 2007 and therefore, the risk of alcohol abuse has dropped, alcohol consumption in Germany remains at a high level, compared to other countries. The proportion of young

---

³ The *Deutscher Werberat* (German Advertising Council) is the self-regulatory body of the advertising industry. The organization ensures that advertising, which is legally permissible, does not exceed ethical boundaries (Deutscher Werberat, 2019, URL).
⁴ According to § 2 *Bürgerliches Gesetzbuch* (German civil code, abbreviated: BGB).

people who regularly drink alcohol has also fallen in the past decade, but is about twice as high with boys than with girls (Drogenbeauftragte der Bundesregierung, 2018, p. 56).

The governance challenge for raising the legal drinking age lies in second-order governance, in the dimension of institutions and organisations. The main task for this topic is to design a new rule and set it up and also implement it accordingly. Another task is the enforcement of such a new rule.

Reduction of economic damage

The economic damage[5] associated with (harmful) alcohol consumption is immense. In the following two figures, several details are laid out and will be explained further down in the section.

The first figure shows the direct cost related to harmful alcohol consumption:

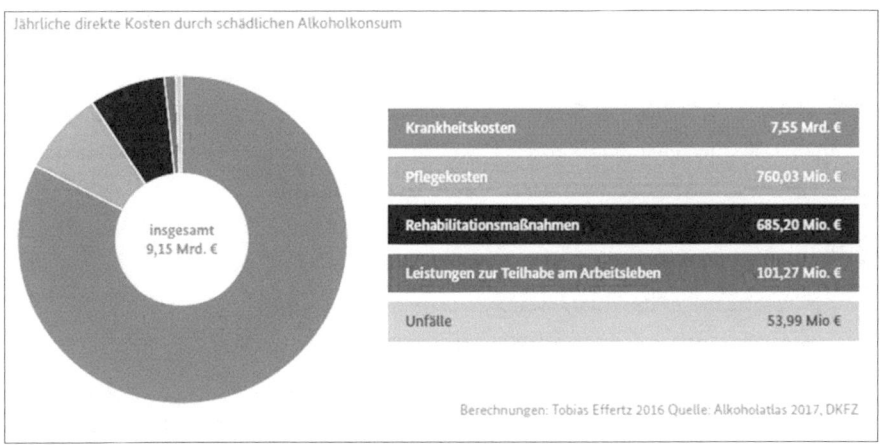

Figure 1 - Direct cost related to harmful alcohol consumption
Source: Schaller, K. et al., 2017, pp. 70; Drogenbeauftragte der Bundesregierung, 2018, p. 70

The major share of the total direct cost of 9.15 bn EUR is made up of *Krankheitskosten* (medical expenses) which include medical treatments, hospitalization, etc. and the minor share of the total direct cost include care, rehabilitation and accidents (Schaller et al., 2017, pp. 70; Drogenbeauftragte der Bundesregierung, 2018, p. 70).

---

[5] The terms 'economic damage' and 'direct / indirect cost' are used synonymous.

The second figure shows the indirect cost related to harmful alcohol consumption:

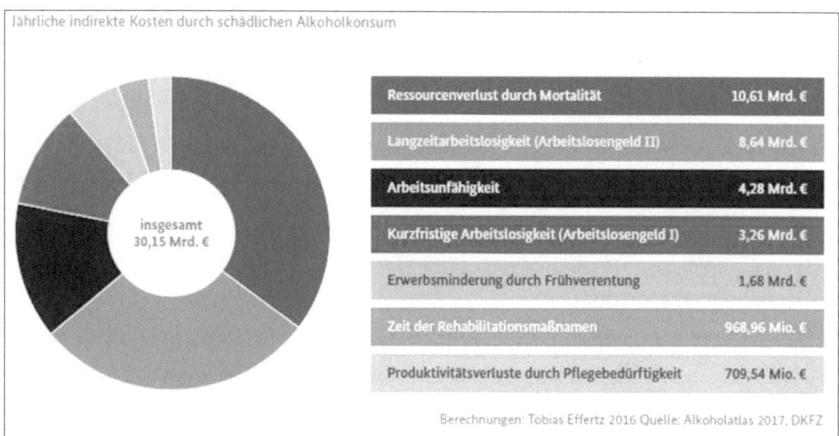

Figure 2 - Indirect cost related to harmful alcohol consumption

Source: Schaller, K. et al., 2017, pp. 70; Drogenbeauftragte der Bundesregierung, 2018, p. 70

Within this figure, the distribution of cost is more differentiated than in Figure 1. The total of 30.15 bn EUR has four major pillars, making up the hugest part of the total indirect costs. The first pillar stands at 10.61 bn EUR and comprises the loss of resources through mortality. The second pillar stands at 8.64 bn EUR and encompasses the long-term unemployment costs. The third pillar stands at 4.28 bn EUR and includes the incapacity of work and the fourth pillar at 3.26 bn EUR comprises of the short-term unemployment costs. The rest of the pillars include early retirement schemes, rehabilitation and cost of care (Schaller et al., 2017, pp. 70; Drogenbeauftragte der Bundesregierung, 2018, p. 70).

The governance challenge for reducing economic damage caused by harmful alcohol consumption lies in second-order governance, in the dimension of institutions and organisations. The main goal would be to design regulations and set up a mode where individual responsibility has to be taken when consuming alcohol in a (harmful) manner, meaning that when certain damages arise, the individual has to take care for itself. This could mean that German national health insurance is not liable when it comes to (harmful) alcohol consumption. This would also mean that the individual has to take measures, e.g. a supplementary insurance, so that the direct or indirect costs and therefore economic damage for the public is reduced.

3 Weakest points of existing interventions

When trying to assess governance performance, three aspects are relevant. The first one is legitimacy of the system as a whole and the key actors, the second one is efficacy of systems and key actors and the third one is effectiveness in ways and means. These three aspects all relate directly to the goal attainment and therefore the performance (Anheier, 2013, pp. 26).

So when trying to figure out the weakest points of existing interventions vis-à-vis the problem of alcohol consumption in Germany, the first aspect to examine is the legitimacy, which is dependent on the adherence to the institutional rules and regulations by actors and authorities on the one hand and on the other hand the trust of those who are affected to uphold these rules an regulations (Anheier, 2013, p. 26). The second aspect is the efficacy, looking at the capacity of those in power and leadership positions, both in a strategical as well as tactical time frame (Anheier, 2013, pp. 26). The third aspect to examine is the effectiveness, trying to figure out the implementation of measures and policies and finding out if the desired results were achieved (Anheier, 2013, p. 27).

Regarding the aspect of legitimacy, the system of addiction prevention in Germany is established and subject of regular evaluation and continued development. Measures of addiction prevention fall under the responsibility of the ministries at federal and state level and are implemented in particular by the *Bundeszentrale für gesundheitliche Aufklärung* (Federal Center for Health Education, abbreviated: BZgA), the federal state level, the municipal level and the self-governing bodies of the insurance carriers (Drogenbeauftragte der Bundesregierung, 2018, p. 10). When examining the efficacy, the federal structure could be criticized. As there are so many actors involved, it is not exactly determined who is doing what. To lay out the differences, it is helpful to provide a structural overview, as laid out by the *DKFZ*, differentiating between *Verhältnisprävention* (conditional prevention) and *Verhaltensprävention* (behavioral prevention). The former is subject to politics and aims at changing the living environment to facilitate behavioral changes for the individual, e.g. via laws and regulations, the latter is subject to many actors like schools, municipalities, national health insurance, etc. and aims at the behavioral change of the individual and the strengthening of the individuals risk competence, e.g. via awareness campaigns or counseling and therapy offerings (Schaller et al., 2017, pp. 76). When assessing the effectiveness, it is necessary to find out if results were achieved with a reasonable amount of effort. The per capita consumption of alcohol has dropped in the last 40 years in Germany. However, compared internationally, Germany continues to be one of the high-consumption countries in the world (Drogenbeauftragte der Bundesregierung, 2018, p. 56). These general remarks still do not allow a specific allocation of results to efforts and for a granular depiction of effective measures, a deeper analysis of efforts has to be made. But based on the aforementioned nearly 40 bn EUR p.a. in economic damage caused through (harmful) alcohol consumption, one could question the effectiveness.

So when considering an effective programme design for tackling the issue, this programme must define the target group and the expected behavior, provide instruments which relate to the behavior as well as an implementation strategy (Mayntz, 1983, p. 127). Two conditions are relevant for effective programmes, first the fit between problem and programme and second the fit between social context and programme design (Cingolani, 2019, p. 11).

Moving further to the standards, it is necessary to determine if it is reasonable to set a rule or a principle. A standard is an "explicit statement about what is prohibited and what is expected and is intended to modify behavior" (Cingolani, 2019, p. 14; Lodge and Wegrich, 2012, pp. 47). A rule is a very clear prescription, lining out an explicit behavior or process. A principle is a broader prescription with the main emphasis on a common goal (Lodge and Wegrich, 2012, pp. 60). As a rule is superior to a principle, especially when subjects need more guidance (Braithwaite, 2002, in Cingolani, 2019, p. 19), in the case of the policy issue in this essay, a rule shall be the choice for the standard.

Picking up the topic of the reduction of economic damages from chapter 2, a possible rule for the policy issue would be a so called self insurance, which would be a financial disincentive for the individual. As pointed out in the previous chapter, this would mean that the individual has to take measures, e.g. a supplementary insurance, so that economic damage for the public is reduced.

4 Delegation of authority

When comparing alcohol consumption on a global level, Europe is the region with the highest consumption worldwide. Regarding risk factors, the consumption of alcohol was the third largest factor for illness and death in the European Union in 2012, after tobacco use and hypertension (Schaller et al., 2017, p. 102). Therefore, the delegation of authority to the supranational level regarding the issue can be a valid approach considering the high relevance for all of the states in Europe.

An argument for the delegation of the issue is the possibility to benefit from expertise on the supranational level and the cooperation with other member states, specifically in this case the delegation to the European Commission. Possible transaction costs through e.g. necessary negotiations could become a challenge, and therefore being a possible counter-argument for delegating authority in the case of this policy issue. The main objectives for delegation are collaboration and coordination (Reh, 2019, pp. 7). As in the specific case of the policy issue in this essay, a certain delegation of authority has already taken place, as pointed out in the according footnotes.[6] [7]

---

[6] In 2017, the European Commission presented a note on the evaluation of the implementation of the EU Drugs Strategy 2013-2020 and the EU Drugs Action Plan 2013-2016. The Commission declared a continued need for the EU Drugs Action Plan 2017-2020. As a result, the Commission has submitted a draft that maintains and strengthens existing measures to address issues which continue to pose a threat to health and safety (Drogenbeauftragte der Bundesregierung, 2018, p. 121).

[7] In 2006, the EU Commission adopted an EU Alcohol Strategy, which was to apply until the end of 2012. For implementation and coordination, the Committee on National Alcohol Policy and Action (CNAPA) and the European Alcohol and Health Forum (EAHF) were established. The CNAPA was set up in 2007 to promote co-operation and coordination between member states and the development of common strategies between member states and with the EU. The committee is composed of national delegations appointed by the member states and holds regular meetings at least twice a year. Its main objectives are the exchange of good practices and the greatest possible alignment of alcohol strategies within the EU. The continuation of the EU Alcohol Strategy was requested by many member states, but at present, despite various decisions, no new alcohol strategy is emerging at European level (Drogenbeauftragte der Bundesregierung, 2018, p. 71).

Bibliography

Course material

Anheier, H. (2013). *Governance – What are the issues?*. Hertie School Governance Report 2013. Berlin, Germany: Oxford University Press

Cingolani, L. (2019). *Rules, principles and financial incentives (Policy Making, CII-1)*. Berlin, Germany

Hertie School (2019). *A quick Hertie School Library guide for EMPA students*. Berlin, Germany

Lodge, M., Wegrich, K. (2012). *Managing Regulation: Regulatory Analysis, Politics and Policy*. Berlin, Germany / London, UK: Red Globe Press

Mayntz, R. (1983). *The Conditions of Effective Public Policy: A New Challenge for Policy Analysis*. Policy & Politics, Volume 11, Number 2, April 1983, pp. 123-143. Bristol, UK: Policy Press

Reh, C. (2019). *Compliance in a Multi-Level Context (Policy Making, CII-1)*. Berlin, Germany

Literature

BSI (2019). *Selbstregulierung von Spirituosen- und Werbebranche*. URL: Link, accessed on November 1st 2019

Deutscher Werberat (2019). *Aufgaben und Ziele*. URL: Link, accessed on November 1st 2019

Deutscher Werberat (2015). *Verhaltensregeln des Deutschen Werberats über die kommerzielle Kommunikation für alkoholhaltige Getränke*. Issued 2009, edited 2015. URL: Link, accessed on November 1st 2019. Berlin, Germany

Drogenbeauftragte der Bundesregierung (2018). *Drogen- und Suchtbericht 2018*. Issued 2018. URL: Link, accessed on November 1st 2019. Berlin, Germany: Druck- und Verlagshaus Zarbock GmbH & Co. KG

Schaller, K. et al. (2017). *Alkoholatlas Deutschland 2017*. Issued 2017. URL: Link, accessed on November 1st 2019. Heidelberg, Germany: Pabst Science Publishers

Singer, M., Teyssen, S. (2001). *Alkohol - Das unterschätzte Gift*. URL: Link, accessed on October 20th 2019

Young, E. (2017). *Suchtprävention - Wie man Jugendliche von Alkohol und Drogen fernhält*. URL: Link, accessed on October 20th 2019

Literature (w/o author)

„Deutschland hat ein Alkoholproblem" (2019). *Jahrbuch Sucht 2019 – Deutschland hat ein Alkoholproblem*. URL: Link, accessed on October 20th 2019

Legal literature

Bundeskinderschutzgesetz (Federal Child Protection Act, abbreviated: BKiSchG)

Jugendschutzgesetz (Protection of Young Persons Act, abbreviated: JuSchG)

Bürgerliches Gesetzbuch (German civil code, abbreviated: BGB)

YOUR KNOWLEDGE HAS VALUE

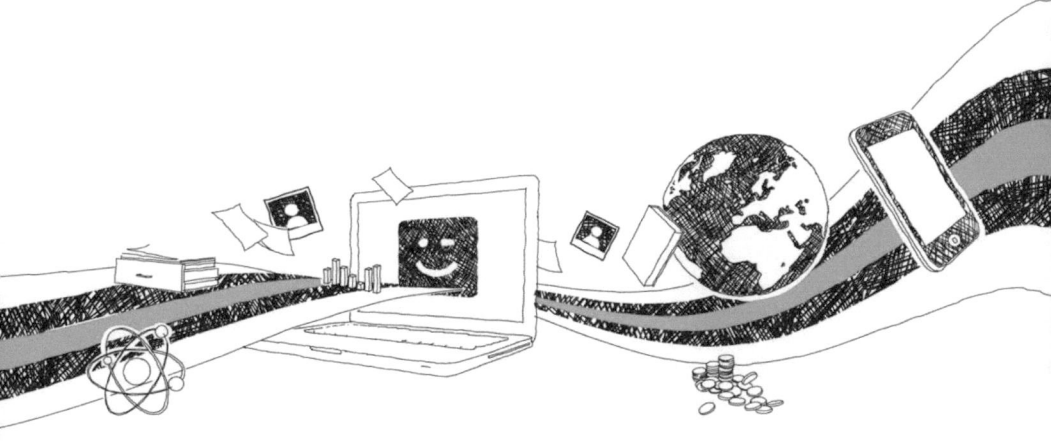

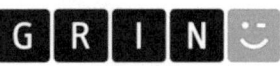